Testimonials for Daniel's Way by Daniel Nardi

"As an Occupational Therapist who has worked with teenagers dealing with mental health issues, I heartily recommend *Daniel's Way*. Daniel has candidly expressed his perspective as an individual with autism spectrum disorder, experiencing depression and anxiety. He also reveals his unique feelings while navigating the mental health system and treatments as he transitioned through adolescence to adulthood. His book is valuable to both those dealing with mental health challenges and their caregivers."

– Lynne Toth OT

"*Daniel's Way* is a personal story of the many trials and tribulations that children and adolescents face following a diagnosis of autism spectrum disorder. I would recommend this book not only to anyone who has suffered from any type of mental illness, but also to those who loved, cared for, and advocated for them."

– Michael R. Nardi PT, DSc, MEd, CMPT

"As a retired psychiatric RN, I truly enjoyed and appreciated reading about Daniel's day-to-day experiences in a variety of mental health settings. Understanding and treating all forms of mental illness is a major problem in this country. I recommend *Daniel's Way* to all health care providers as well as anyone suffering from mental health issues. Thank you, Daniel, for sharing your story."

– Kathryn K. VanDresser RN

Daniel's Way

Daniel's Way

Exploring My Experiences with ASD and Mental Health

DANIEL NARDI

Copyright © 2021 by Daniel Nardi.

All rights reserved. No part of this book may be reproduced or transmitted in any form or by any means, electronic or mechanical, including photocopying, recording, or by any information storage or retrieval system, without written permission from the author or the publisher, except for the inclusion of brief quotations in a review.

Published by Cincinnati Book Publishing – Cincinnati, Ohio
www.CincyBooks.com

Anthony W. Brunsman, president
Sue Ann Painter, executive editor
Alaina Stellwagen, associate editor
Kayla Stellwagen, layout design

Softbound ISBN: 978-1-7355873-6-3
E-Book ISBN: 978-1-7355873-7-0
Library of Congress Control Number: 2021931276
Printed in the United States of America

First Edition, 2021

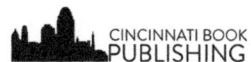

DANIEL NARDI

Daniel's Way

My Experiences with ASD
and Mental Health

Cincinnati Book Publishing
Cincinnati, Ohio

Contents

Acknowledgements   1

Introduction   3

Chapter One: Early Age Story: Sandusky   5

Chapter Two: The Start: Accommodating
the Special Needs   9

Chapter Three: Inpatient/Outpatient: My Orientation to
Cincinnati Children's Medical + Psychiatric Treatment   13

Chapter Four: 2SW: Children's College Hill Psychiatric Unit   21

Chapter Five: Last Resort: Electroconvulsive Therapy (ECT)   33

Chapter Six: One Year Update: May 2020   39

Chapter Seven: Depression and Suicide: The Reality   45

Chapter Eight: Mental Health: Positive Coping Skills   49

Chapter Nine: Set Back: September 2020   51

Chapter Ten: A Mother's Perspective – Julie Nardi   55

Chapter Eleven: ASD: Signs/Symptoms/
Diagnosing and Treatment   59

Support Services   63

Sources   65

Acknowledgements

I want to thank my father, Michael Nardi PT, DSc, MEd, CMPT, and my mother, Julie Nardi MSN, RN, for supporting me with their financial, spiritual, and emotional support throughout my many years of emotional ups and downs. I also want to acknowledge those people who have assisted in the production of *Daniel's Way* through their financial contributions. Dr. Michael and Julie Nardi, Richard Nardi, Stephen Bartow, Julia Bouzaher, Michael Bond, Edward and Sylvia Gembka (my grandparents), Sydney Gembka, Ed and Sandra Gembka, Amy McDuffie, Perry Denehy, Alisha Smith, Linda Waters, Kathryn VanDresser, Melanie Etheridge: Without your contributions, this book may not have been published. So, I thank you very much.

I would like to give a very sincere thank you to the teachers and counselors at Sycamore High School, the staff on 2SW at Cincinnati Children's Hospital Medical Center at the College Hill Campus, friends that I have worked with in Project SEARCH, my managers and mentors, the Montgomery and Loveland Police Departments, IKRON Corporation, and the many therapists and doctors who cared for me.

Introduction

There's a road in life that eventually comes to an end. It's up to you to decide the path you wish to follow. My path began when I was diagnosed with autism spectrum disorder (ASD) at age 3. I grew up functioning at a high level and many people questioned my diagnoses. I never wanted anyone to know that I had ASD because I felt it could ruin my relationships or informal encounters throughout my time in school and everywhere I stepped foot.

As I got older and graduated from high school, I began to tell people I was suffering from ASD. Many said, "You're very high functioning for someone who has ASD." I would reply, "Yes, but do you know there are many different signs/symptoms and severity of ASD?" Personally, I began to understand the diagnosis was correct, while realizing that my disorder was mild. I will always need help in certain areas. For those who interact with someone with ASD, it is important to realize that the afflicted person isn't necessarily ignoring you or not paying attention. I am a quiet person, and I often struggle with communication and social cues, which is a symptom of ASD.

When I first became aware that I had ASD, I looked it up on Google. I was surprised because I've never heard of it before. I didn't think anything was seriously wrong with me, although I was having difficulty communicating and learning. I knew something could be wrong, but I had difficulty accepting the diagnoses. Then, I noticed some other areas within myself that were different, and I realized those symptoms were part of ASD. Some of these areas were failure to make eye contact, hypersensitivity to lights and noise, and trouble with memorization, social skills, reading and writing, and behavioral issues.

I am now 20 years old and have experienced depression, anxiety, multiple medication changes, inpatient/outpatient mental health treatment, and even ECT. I have struggled for many years wondering if I would be better off dead. Suicidal ideation has been the hardest challenge for me and my family.

In the following chapters I will detail my personal experience coming to grips with this disorder, and how it manifested into anxiety and major depression. Lastly, I will also discuss the current research and treatment of ASD. My hope is that the readers who struggle with this disorder will benefit from my personal experiences.

Chapter One
Early Age Story: Sandusky

I was born in Sandusky, Ohio, and lived there the first eight years of my life. It is the only place that has truly felt like home because I noticed different aspects of the environment there as compared to Cincinnati. The air feels different, the people are much nicer, the school systems are much different, and the jazz music on 107.3 The Wave is special. Sandusky is a small town, unlike Cincinnati. I lived in a nice house and my neighbors were considered close friends. There was a vibe that can't be found anywhere else, and I felt like Sandusky was that place. My father had his own practice, called Advanced Health, right down the road and my mother was at home to help raise her children. At times, when I hear a radio playing, I remember Sandusky—just the feeling of being in that town. I recall feelings of calmness, happiness, and joyfulness. Most of my family grew up in Northern Ohio. My mother grew up in Huron and my grandpa and grandma grew up in Elyria/Lorain/Amherst.

I grew up on a street called Autumn Ridge Lane in Sandusky. I know every part of that neighborhood till this day. Friends right across the street, the sledding hill, and the shortcut to another neighborhood. Not only did I enjoy my own neighborhood, but I enjoyed Sandusky. I visited friends over on Lake Erie, on Cedar Point Drive, and I would sail with my brothers and friends on Lake Erie. I walked around the Sandusky Mall and visited my grandparents who were right down the road. I went to Cedar Point amusement park and Kalahari water park, which were only ten minutes from where I lived. My mother would take us to visit Huron and get ice cream at Pied Piper.

In the summer, usually in late June, which is very close to my birthday, my family would rent a house on Kelley's Island or we would go camping on a piece of land across from the cemetery. If we were staying in the house, which was directly across the street from Lake Erie, we would rent a golf cart for the week. Driving in the golf cart was so much fun! The sky was blue. The air was fresh, although sometimes it would smell like dead fish. As kids, we could do whatever we wanted to. Most often, my aunt would come and stay with us too. They would pack coolers and we would drive to the state park to play on the beach all day. I would try to catch the little minnows swimming in the surf with my net and bucket. My mom would bring the sunscreen often because I was very focused on catching the fish, unaware that I might get a sunburn. After a day at the beach, we went home, cleaned up, and went out to dinner. The sunsets were so beautiful. We sat on the beach on our old beach blanket with a bonfire, making smores. For one whole week this is what we did.

I loved to go fishing. Still to this day, I look forward to fishing with my dad. I may only catch a small fish on the lake in Vermont, but just being with him and throwing the line in the water brings back memories. We also fish in the Gulf of Mexico with friends and catch much larger fish.

Another time, when we were camping on Kelly's Island, my dad brought us over on the sailboat. I had to wear the big orange life preserver and I was scared of getting seasick. We rented a golf cart and set up camp. During the morning we drove around then stopped for lunch. Mom was taking a rest and I guess she thought I was going to as well. However, I was so focused on fishing I just took my pole and left. I walked two miles into town. I did not tell my dad and my brothers, who were off hiking in Quarry. I really wanted to fish, and our friend was due to arrive at the dock at any time. I wanted to meet him at the dock to go fishing. I was only six-years-old at the time. Our friend saw me there by myself and thankfully brought me back home. My mom was so happy that I did not fall in the lake.

As time went on, I developed more interests. I tried soccer at one point. I did not like soccer and had a difficult time with team sports. However, when I was playing with my brothers, I was often the goalie for their street hockey games. I suited up with a mask and pads, ready to take on whatever shot came. I was very good at focusing on one thing such as the ball or the puck. When roller hockey came around at the local skating rink, I was signed up as goalie and played the whole year.

I also did well in swimming—freestyle and backstroke were my forte. I excelled at team sports with an individual component. I did not like the contact aspect of hockey, as physical contact is an issue for me. With swimming, I did well until we had to compete in the finals in an indoor venue. The noise from the buzzer and all the cheering was too much for me to manage. One of the symptoms of autism is sensory overload. My family has recognized this and has tried to control this. Hearing, touching, tasting are senses which are heightened for me. Hearing has benefited me and provided me with the ability to sing on tune.

I have learned how to look people in the eye when I am speaking to them. This has been challenging in the past. When I played sports, my coaches wanted me to look at them when they spoke to me, not knowing why I had such a difficult time doing that. Early on I felt very uncomfortable with eye contact but have learned how important eye contact is when communicating.

I enjoy many different types of foods. This is most likely related to the fact that I can taste many variations of spices and concoctions, appreciating all the combinations. My mother would often say I could smell her perfume from a mile away. I knew the minute she arrived home and I would be running down the stairs to see her, day or night.

The sense of touch has been a major challenge for me. It is one that brought my preschool teacher to alert my mother to have me tested for autism. The teacher told my mother I would sit by the girl with long brown hair and pet her hair. Not long after that was when I was diagnosed. When our neighbor had a garage sale, I found a mink fur collar at the sale and the neighbor gave it to me because I sat and stroked it all day. Like many other individuals with ASD, physical touch is very difficult and often unwanted. This has been a challenge in the past, coming from an Italian and Polish upbringing.

Chapter Two
The Start: Accommodating the Special Needs

When I was three-years-old, I was diagnosed with autism. From an early age I would have a hard time communicating how I felt, which would lead me to become upset and agitated. I learned how to walk and talk later than most children. When I turned six, I attended preschool, and I was very active in my education plan. My mother would make sure that I was doing well in school. I would attend classes where I would learn how to read and write. I remember a time when my mother took me out into the hall, and I was crying. I knew that my life was difficult even at an early age.

When I began formal education, I was given an IEP (Individualized Education Plan). This plan would help me throughout my school years, and I was given accommodations such as extended time on tests or given oral exams. I would go to different places within the school to take a test or work on homework. My IEP was structured to help me be successful and graduate. Most of my teachers understood what an IEP was and how it should be used to help me succeed. Generally, I did well in school, but I had some difficulties with certain subjects. These subjects included English, history, mathematics, and biology. I would never fail a class in school, but I was not learning. I was focused on getting good grades because I didn't want to be a failure.

As I entered middle school, I began to learn more and more about myself and my ASD. I wasn't able to pick up on reading and writing at an early age. However, with help over time, I became more fluent and vocal. I felt more comfortable with myself when I started middle school although I continued to have problems with communication and social interaction.

I was very active throughout my elementary and middle school days. In fourth grade I began to play basketball and made many friends. For the first time I felt like I belonged and had friends. I tried out and made the A team for basketball in middle school. I practiced every day for hours trying to get better and improve my skills on the court and off the court as well.

As time went on, I played for the school basketball team and many club teams leading up to high school. When I entered high school, I tried out my freshmen year and made the team. I felt connected and met new people who guided me along a positive path.

I was involved in competitive basketball my freshmen year and learned how to be a member of the team. I got yelled at and had to pick myself up every day in practice. Many times, I almost passed out from the conditioning drills. I knew that later on in high school I wanted to continue basketball, but I didn't like what came with it. I was debating whether to give basketball up or fight hard to get myself a spot on the team.

In my sophomore year, I became more quiet and shy. I didn't really speak up for myself. I wanted to fit in and speak with new people, but most times I didn't know how to initiate conversations. I just wanted to be by myself. I isolated myself from people, and I didn't like large gatherings.

As I entered my junior year, I started to notice a dark and sad feeling, like a dark cloud was over me everywhere I walked. I was able to make it to the third quarter of school and then, all of a sudden, I crashed. I experienced my first admission to the children's psychiatric hospital and was in the hospital for about a week. Once I got out, I competed the fourth quarter by homeschooling and working on papers that needed to be done. With the help of my teacher, Mrs. Oltorik, I was successfully able to complete my junior year. I cut off many of my friends and didn't respond or communicate with anyone other than my teachers. I feel as if I ignored and left relationships behind. I knew that my senior year was going to be a challenge, knowing that I had major depression symptoms.

Once I got to my senior year of high school, I was a complete mess. I'd already experienced my first couple hospitalizations. When I was out of the hospital, I was transported to Aves Academy, which was at the Blue Ash Elementary, where I would continue with my senior year online through apex. I missed about 70 days of my senior year of high school. I was sad, angry, frustrated, and most importantly, I felt like my life was over.

CHAPTER TWO

You never know what life will lead to. I never thought tragedies would happen to me. I never thought I'd be put through traumatic events. I never thought I'd miss my senior year. I never thought I would have major depression.

Chapter Three

Inpatient/Outpatient: My Orientation to Cincinnati Children's Medical + Psychiatric Treatment

Let's take a step back to my high school experiences. As I entered my sophomore year of high school, I decided to stop playing basketball, and I threw away my chance of playing on the basketball team. Instead, I joined the ice hockey team. I've always wanted to play with my brother, who was the captain of the ice hockey team. I knew that this was my chance to fulfill that dream. My brother was a senior and this was his last year of ice hockey. I skated with my brother—that was one of the greatest experiences of my life. Till this day I knew that playing ice hockey with my brother instead of playing on the basketball team was the best decision I've made. Although I met people through basketball, I gained more relationships through ice hockey as well.

In high school, my grades were up to par, and I was meeting expectations. I knew that I was on the right track to graduating. I didn't do so well on test taking. I was beginning to fail, and I knew that there was something inside of me that wasn't right. As I entered my junior year of high school, I began to notice that I was feeling increasingly sad. Many days I walked around school crying. I began to lose friendships and my brother was not in school with me anymore. I wasn't hanging around the right people.

I felt like I was being ignored and I felt guilty. I felt numb and was always thinking about taking my life. I can't feel the pain as much anymore, but I still have a feeling within my body that I remember when I tried to take my life.

I didn't try out for basketball or ice hockey my junior year. I wasn't involved in any sports or clubs. I felt alone, lonely, and very depressed. My grades were suffering along with my personal life.

During my class instruction, I often had to leave class to talk with my counselor and school psychologist. My mother would often come pick me up from school early. Most days I walked into school for an hour or two, then had to leave due to my depression and anxiety. I went to the bathroom almost every day to journal or call my mother. I walked out of school a couple times and started walking home. My depression was getting worse and my doctors prescribed different antidepressants. Most of the medication I took wasn't helping. My medication was getting switched around so much to the point where I began to notice that I was having increased suicidal ideation.

My life took a turn quickly. I was admitted to Cincinnati Children's Hospital for the first time during my junior year. I went to see my doctor and I mentioned that I just wanted to end my life. I was preparing for what was the worst to come. I was taken to the emergency room and I became agitated, throwing clothes around. I was causing a scene right there on the unit.

Eventually, security was called up to where I was and told me to return to my patient room. I wasn't following any directions and then I started to fight. I came after the staff and they all held me down. I was put in restraints on a hospital bed. My legs and arms were locked down to the bed and I couldn't do anything. I was trying to break out of the restraints that were holding me down. I almost flipped the bed. If I had, I would've hurt myself really bad. This experience was very traumatic for me and my family.

I was given two pills of Zyprexa, which helped me feel relaxed and calm. I fell asleep and woke up feeling better. I knew that later on I made poor decisions and that I should've just followed through in the emergency room so that I could've been taken home. Instead, I ended up in a position I didn't want to be in. My journey throughout hospitalizations had just begun.

The next day I was taken to the Children's College Hill campus where I was put on the unit, 3 South West (3SW). This was the first of my five admissions. I was admitted for agitation. I was introduced to my mental health specialists (MHS), Mr. Okama and Mrs. Amber. I had no idea what I was supposed to do in the hospital or what direction I was headed in. The unit I was on housed patients who were lower functioning than me and non-verbal. I was thinking in my head,

CHAPTER THREE

"Where am I, and why am I here?" I put on the hospital clothes and got settled in. I almost punched one of the MHS. I squared up and was waiting for the MHS to swing. I calmed down and returned to my room. I never thought too much about how long I was going to stay. I was just yelling, "Let me go home." When I woke up the next day, Mr. Okama took me down to the basketball court that was inside the hospital. This was my first time hanging out with Mr. Okama. I never got a chance to meet other staff. One night on the unit, I woke up and I felt like I've had enough, so I walked out of my room and said, "Who's ready to fight?" and I was about to attack one of the staff. I ended up calming down and went back into my room. I was discharged from the hospital a couple days later when the insurance limits were met. My first admission wasn't due to my depression, but it was concentrated on my agitation and how to handle becoming upset because I came after some people and I was out of control.

After I was discharged, I returned home. However, my depression was unchanged. I landed back in the emergency room a couple months later. I was still in my junior year, homeschooling. I was admitted to the Children's College Hill campus yet again.

During my second admission I was on the unit, 3 North (3N). This time I was with patients on the unit who didn't have disabilities or any special needs. I was taken onto the unit and when I entered, the patients were staring at me and I felt intimidated. Later on, I became connected with these patients, nurses (RN), and mental health specialists (MHS). I attended groups and I learned a lot during this admission. I was interacting a lot with the patients on the unit. I was laughing and, at some point, having a good time with my fellow patients and staff. Some of my fellow patients would mess around and weren't really focused on treatment. I was included in the messing around and I was having a good time when really, I should've been focused on my treatment plan. On the unit, we played games with our MHS and nurses. This was not what I expected. Although I had a good time, I learned new coping skills, how to recognize and manage my triggers, and breathing exercises that helped me feel better. I had a folder where I kept the papers that I had to fill out. If I ever wanted to go off the unit then I would have to complete the papers in my folder. I attended groups and became more familiar with the unit. My doctor was still moving my medications around, and would check me every so often to monitor my depression and anxiety.

During my stay, I went off the unit and played basketball with the patients in an inside basketball court that was part of the hospital. When I went off the unit for the first time, I saw other patients. One of the staff, Mr. Brandon, took me to play 3-on-3 basketball with other patients as well. I had met Mr. Brandon way before my stay on 2SW. He came around to take me off the unit and hang out with me. Mr. Brandon took me off the unit one time to go to a drawing class. I had my own notebook and I would draw in it. The staff was excited to see what I could draw. I remember it was October 2018 when I was in the hospital, so I would draw Halloween pictures. The other patients there were artists as well.

I became connected with the patients and although being in the hospital is not a pleasant experience, I still found a way to get around my depression and focus on being in the moment. I didn't think I was going to hurt myself, so one week later, I was discharged. I got in the car to go home and it felt like I'd never been in a car before. I'd sat in the hospital watching time go by on the clock outside of my room. It just seemed like I was in the hospital for a long time, but it was only for 11 days.

I went to the high school and talked with some of my teachers. I kept saying that I was fine when in reality, I was still depressed and anxious. I walked into one of my teachers' rooms and they all knew that I have been absent for two weeks. They asked if I was ok, and I said yes. I was continuing to homeschool. I tried to get a key to the medication box so I could overdose on prescription pills. I wasn't able to get in the box but then a couple days later my mother found out and decided to have me admitted again, this time to the unit, 3 South (3S). I was introduced to new MHS and new patients. This time, I stayed for 17 days. I was attending groups and following hospital guidelines. We played games on the unit and when we had groups we had to participate. The staff started to notice that my heart rate was 40 bpm. Over time my heartrate got better but during my stay I noticed that it was concerning. I said that I was feeling better and my social worker agreed. I actually wasn't really feeling well this admission. I was then discharged and sent back home, hoping that I'd never have to come back.

My depression began to really take control of my life. Throughout my admissions I was so focused on wanting to go home that I didn't really work towards helping with my depression. I was to follow up with outpatient therapy when I was discharged, where I attended a partial day program in Green Township through Cincinnati Children's. I went to the program from 8 a.m. until 4 p.m. I met new patients again and I worked with new MHS and nurses. We had groups, played games, and watched videos. I learned a lot about my depression and suicidal ideation. I felt connected with my fellow patients all through the partial program and through my inpatient stay at College Hill. I went to the partial program for a week. I had a meeting with my teachers, and they all wanted me to complete some papers and tests so that I would complete my credits for all my classes during my junior year. I worked with Mrs. Oltorik, and she was very helpful. I was expected to finish out homeschooling, which I did.

I would leave school often and when I was admitted, some of my friends would ask where I was because I never showed up to school. I told my friends that I was in the hospital. Some were worried about me. I just told my friends that I was struggling mentally. Now, if you're my friend and you're reading, then you know why I wasn't at school. Many people found out that I tried to end my life. I was not allowed to have my phone on me when I was inpatient but when I was discharged from the hospital, I received many text messages.

After discharge from inpatient therapy at College Hill I was referred to outpatient at Green Township. I was allowed to bring my phone in, but I would keep it somewhere where I couldn't use it. At Green Township, I would have time to participate and play games. I met Mr. Ron, who was a MHS. He would have us play a game where you would have to roll dice and get a certain number. I liked hanging out with Mr. Ron—he was very helpful and supportive. I would attend outpatient therapy from 8 a.m. until 4 p.m. for a week and sometimes more. When I arrived at 8 a.m., the staff would bring out breakfast, such as cereal, juice, and fruits, on a tray. I didn't enjoy the food, but I ate anyway because I needed food in my system. Later on, in the day I would draw, paint, and I was encouraged to participate in groups. When I was an inpatient at Cincinnati Children's Hospital, I attended daily groups. These groups were very important for me to attend as they were considered part of my treatment. The groups were helpful because they helped me structure my day and develop goals to work toward.

Some groups were led by an individual such as a mental health specialist or a music teacher who brings items to let us (in the group) to discuss or play instruments. Many groups are open discussions where patients discussed subjects such as depression or anxiety.

As an inpatient, participating in these group sessions not only helped me get better, but the practice was counted toward my being eligible for discharge.

As an outpatient, I also attended groups such as the Getting Out Of Depression group (GOOD). While an outpatient at Cincinnati Children's Green Township location, I participated in groups that focused on art and music. I also learned other helpful practices such as Cognitive Behavioral Therapy (CBT), mindfulness, and deep breathing exercises. The lazy-eight breathing and six sides of breathing are two techniques in breathing exercises that I learned.

All groups I attended and still attend, are very important. They help me feel better mentally and physically. Group sessions help make me more aware and able to cope with my diagnosis of major depression, as well as ASD.

Some of the groups consisted of Cognitive Behavioral Therapy, speech group, and art group. For the first time I started to learn new coping skills and put them into practice. For example, when I got agitated, I would use a breathing exercise. When I was feeling depressed, I would watch movies, videos, and I would listen to music. I had a new scale from 1-10 on how depressed I was feeling. That scale was updated as

CHAPTER THREE

I was an outpatient. I was first introduced to the scale in high school by Mrs. Collins, who was my special education teacher and as time went on, I used the scale more often. When in outpatient therapy, there was lunch time and just like when I was inpatient at College Hill, I would fill out a paper with a marker for what I wanted to have for lunch the next day. I would end the day off at Green Township by filling out a paper that included questions such as, what coping skill did you learn today, or what will you do differently tomorrow? After I filled out the paper, I would wait for my mother, father, or brother to come pick me up so that I could return home.

Chapter Four
2SW: Children's College Hill Psychiatric Unit

As I entered my senior year of high school, I still felt depressed. I was recommended for online classes in which I attended Aves Academy. My first day went well and I was feeling comfortable. After a couple days passed, I started to feel suicidal. I told my mother that I needed to go back to the hospital. I was admitted yet again to the Children's College Hill campus. I was admitted to the unit 2 South West (2SW). I was on the unit with patients who were lower functioning, but there were also patients who came in that I was able to communicate with. I was on the unit for a week before I met with my doctor and my care manager.

I finally met with the rehabilitation team and it was recommended that I stay longer to figure out how I could stop myself from wanting to commit suicide and how to manage my depression. At the beginning of my stay, I had no idea how long I was going to stay. I honestly thought it was going to be one or two weeks and then I'd be discharged. Instead, after meeting with the rehab team, the recommendation was to consider a treatment called electro convulsive therapy (ECT). I was upset and filled with many emotions. I thought my life was over. At the time, I didn't realize I could overcome this challenge and make it out. When in reality, Mrs. Emily reminded me that my time in the hospital was only temporary. I was very agitated, and I went to my room and started to break down. I was in my room laying on my bed yelling, "I don't know what I'm going to do," for an hour. This was the saddest I've ever been, and I was told that this was my only option because medication was not working.

This admission was my longest and my stay lasted 50 days. I met and worked with so many different people that it was hard to keep track of my treatment plan. My first day on the unit, my MHS, Mr. Okama, walked in my room. I knew I'd seen him before during my first admission, which was a year before. This time, I would become connected with Mr. Okama throughout my stay. The first thing Mr. Okama and I talked about was why I returned. Mr. Okama said,

"You look like a very nice man without any problems." There are many people in this world who live in poverty and don't have what I have. At that time, I didn't realize how blessed I was, and that I just needed to get past this illness. Mr. Okama always had my back and although we don't communicate anymore, I still consider him one of my favorite people because, during the worst part of my life, he was there for me. I will always have a special place in my heart for Mr. Okama.

After my first day on the unit, Mr. Okama introduced me to Mr. Shawn and I later met more people like Mrs. Amber and Ms. Maggie and the list goes on. I worked with many people who were all supportive and helpful. Everyone on the unit made an effort to have positive communications with me. They hated to see me depressed and they all wanted me to be successful.

I knew that the staff I had was special and unique. I would never be able to find people like I did on that unit. Most of the staff understood me and when I got angry or sad, they helped me cool down and work through the issues that I was having. One day I got upset and ripped stuff off the wall. Mrs. Cheryl had made a monthly calendar that I was about to tear off the wall, but I was able to calm down, realizing that it was there to help me. During my stay, I tore up many things and destroyed property due to my agitation. I struggled to control my agitation but would often calm down and return to my room.

Whenever I got upset, I would pace around the unit and would try to open the door and escape. I was rejected to go off the unit sometimes because of my actions and behaviors. My doctors and staff wanted to make sure I was being safe. At some points I was not being safe and would try to start fights. As time went on, I thought more and more about ECT, which fueled my agitation.

I never agreed to ECT treatment. I thought that the treatment would ruin my life and I didn't want to get ketamine and IVs in my arm. I was told that I would have mini seizures during the treatment. I thought that ECT was the wrong choice and I refused to have the treatment.

While in my room with my laptop, I would go on YouTube and look up ECT. I was upset to see what the treatment was, and I would express how I felt about this treatment with my staff. My staff would tell me that some of the videos were not really what the treatment would be like. The videos were just scaring me, and I knew that I did not want to go through this treatment.

I would also look up new medications that I would be taking. When I saw the side effects that could come with the medication, I became very concerned. I would later on experience tremors from weaning off the medication. I couldn't control my behavior; I was shaking every day, and the patients on the unit made it worse because they were yelling every second of the day. Some patients would run around the unit and jump onto the wall next to my room. It would piss me off because I was just trying to sleep or lay down and watch TV.

Because of my increased agitation, I almost got involved in fights when I was on different units. One patient thought I was staring at him, so he came in my room and told me to square up. I didn't expect him to get in my face, so I told him to back up. A couple seconds later he left my room and the staff shut my door.

On 2SW I didn't really experience fights, but the unit would call a code violet, which was announced throughout the hospital when a patient is in danger or a danger to others. On the unit I would hear code violet a lot, and I saw a patient on the unit that was put in restraints. There were a couple of code blues. Code blue is when a patient needs medical help. When I was sleeping, I would wake up to not only the loud patients, but a code red, which was an alarm that would play if there was a fire or a fire drill, throughout the building. I would get very mad and frustrated because I was trying to sleep and every time I went to bed, something would wake me up out of my sleep.

Prior to prescribing ECT treatments I attended probate court. I wrote, "Today I woke up and was ready for court. The officers came a little late to pick me up." (9/28/18) I got into a black police van and the police took me to court. I had to take the shoelaces out of my shoes and be escorted out safely.

Once I got to court, I waited in a small area with patients from different hospitals who were older than me. One man told me, "Your life matters, you're so young, I would do the time for you." One of the patients was out of control. The patients weren't mentally right, and they were worse than me. It was difficult to see these patients as they were. When they called my name, I came into the courtroom. I met with an attorney before I entered court. I told him that I didn't want ECT. He said, "Do you know why you're here? You tried to commit suicide." I didn't like what he had to say. I was in the courtroom for ten minutes.

I would ride in the back of a police van, and while we drove to probate court I was thinking about my life, how I had messed up, and what I could've done differently. I didn't expect to go to court during my stay. I would appear in court twice. My first court appearance involved conversations about my signature to leave the hospital. I didn't want to spend any more time in the hospital. Dr. Lemy had me sign a slip of paper saying that I want to be discharged. My second court appearance was for my refusal for the ECT treatment. The magistrate signed a piece of paper saying that I would be required to get ECT. Before my second appearance, I wrote a note about what I was going to say in court. Although my attorney told me I shouldn't say anything, I read my note.

Once I got back from court, I met with Mr. Shawn and we went to the rec room and played pool. I remember I turned on the song, "Heartless," by Kanye West. Mr. Shawn and I had common interests. We like the same music and we like to draw and write. Mr. Shawn liked comic books and Spiderman. I learned so many new things during my stay and I left this time feeling better. Mr. Shawn brought in his PlayStation, which was the coolest thing. I got to play on a PlayStation in the hospital. I knew this stay was way different from the others because I was given more freedom in the choice of activities.

I wouldn't have to fill out as much paperwork as I did on the other units. I was more independent and responsible. Mrs. Amber would have me keep good hygiene. I wouldn't brush my teeth some days and she would tell me how important it is to have good hygiene. I just liked to mess around and laugh but some stuff was serious. I needed to take care of myself. Depression left me numb and discouraged me from doing the important things in life.

CHAPTER FOUR

When I was an inpatient, I would have a difficult time using the restroom. I wouldn't go for days and the most days I spent without using the restroom was 14 days. I felt like I couldn't have any privacy because I was being watched all the time. I would take medication to help me go such as Miralax, Senna, prune juice, and Metamucil. All these medications were in me two weeks and my stomach got bigger because I had so much built up in me. One day I finally went and the whole unit was relieved that I finally went. I just thought the whole situation was funny and people were surprised that I didn't go to the bathroom for two weeks. Some situations were serious and personally, I wasn't serious at all. I still managed to make it out and I'm here today.

One day I woke up feeling agitated. I was thinking about being in the hospital for so long and the pending ECT treatments. I came out of my room and started to yell and cuss at Mr. Okama and others. My agitation was at an all-time high. I was so angry but then I began to break down again, crying in my bed. I just wanted to go home.

When I was on the unit, my day would consist of attending groups. One of the groups was music therapy. I remember the music lady brought instruments and I played with my group. I played a banjo, the piano, a guitar, and drums. The music therapy lady brought me a computer privately at times and I worked in a program called Garage Band. I put together a beat.

My favorite instrument was the piano. I was playing on the keys and everyone liked what I was playing. I felt great when I was playing instruments. I also played drums and when I make beats, I use drums. I felt like I was in my own studio at home playing with these types of instruments. I hadn't felt that feeling in a while.

Personally, I love music, especially making music. I work in music Daws such as Pro Tools 12 and FL Studio. I knew all about different kinds of music. I realized that music was extremely therapeutic for me.

Also, during my stay, I would request what I would like for breakfast, lunch, and dinner. I filled out a paper every morning with a marker. I did not like the food. I thought it was funny when Mr. Okama would place the tray with a cover on the table and once he took the cover off, the food looked disgusting. We were laughing and I said, "Get that out of my face." So, I requested a cheeseburger many times when I didn't like the food I was given. Mr. Okama came through with what I wanted.

I was brought a laptop to work on my online classes for Aves Academy. If I wanted to graduate, I was required to finish and earn all my credits. I remember I had a personal finance class through Apex, which is an online program. The class was difficult, and I was struggling. I asked for help and most of the workers I was with on the unit were struggling as well to help me with that assignment. I remember Mr. Ben started helping me and then all of a sudden, the whole unit was trying to figure out the math problem. I wrote, "Today I continue to work on math and the staff can't figure it out." (10/4/18)

I also got to watch TV in my room. I would keep the same channel on other than when I watched movies. I watched sports channels whenever I was in my room. I watched a movie called "Million Dollar Arm" about 15 times throughout my stay.

On the unit, you could hear the TVs from every patient's room and the TVs that were on would play the "Liberty, liberty, liberty, liberty" commercial and the "Despicable Me" soundtrack. I remember I would play music from my laptop I had for my schoolwork. I like all kinds of music, so I would play different types of music and staff were surprised that I knew the music I was playing.

I was filled with so many emotions during my stay. Some good and bad. I felt like I was never going to make it out of this depression. One day I wrote, "I have never felt so down in my life. I failed. I gave up on myself." (10/7/18) I thought my whole life was going to change, and I wouldn't make it out in a good way. I felt really bad that I missed numerous days of school and still graduated. I needed help, and at the end of the day, I got it.

I was able to attend daily groups on the unit. There would be an ice breaker, such as, "What is your favorite sports team with the

CHAPTER FOUR

letter C?" I would also talk about my goal for the week such as, "Managing my anger" or "Writing in my journal." Many of the patients on the unit were non-verbal but there were some patients that came through and were communicating with me. I saw patients come and go on the unit just like the other units I've stayed on. 2SW was the unit I will remember the most because of the relationships I built and how I got to learn more about myself, working with the staff and even the patients.

I became familiar with the hospital. I was held on different units and I went different places within the hospital. I liked hanging out with staff but the reason I was there was to get help, which I did.

I personally don't think I will be able to go back and visit the unit because of the hospital policies, such as the HIPAA law and confidentiality. On the unit, there were rules that I had to follow. Some of them, I broke. Rules like, maintaining good hygiene, attending groups, and many more. One rule that I broke was attempting to escape from the unit, which negatively impacted me by not being able to go off the unit for a week and not being able to go close to the door. I was being watched 24/7. I didn't necessarily like that I was on suicide watch because I wanted privacy. I learned more rules and policies throughout my stay.

I turned 18-years-old during my stay. I thought I could make my own decisions, but my parents disagreed and filed for legal guardianship. I was treated like an adult and I got more privileges. I was expected to make the right decisions. At the time, I was not making good decisions. I continued to have suicidal ideation, which resulted in having privileges taken away from me. The loss increased my agitation.

Even though I continued to struggle with depression, I tried to follow my treatment plan. When you're put in a tough situation, you have to make the best of it. I knew my MHS and nurses were always there for me and cared about me.

In some groups, I would be the only verbal patient. The staff spent a great deal of time talking with me. I would feel too old for certain things, but I still participated. Some of the groups included smelling certain fruits, music, and exercise. Mrs. Amber brought out a TV that had "Just Dance" on the Wii. I would dance and get the highest score. I felt really good participating, and Mrs. Amber made sure that I was smiling. My vertical jump was decent, and I was able to jump up and touch the ceiling. Mrs. Amber was impressed that I was able to do that. One thing I miss about Mrs. Amber is that she was nice and considerate; I felt a strong connection with her.

On the unit, I spent my time with not only the staff but patients. These patients I spent time with were mostly lower functioning and had difficulty doing things on their own. Some of the patients were very loud and I went to bed and woke up every morning with someone yelling and screaming. I got so angry one night that I got up out of my bed and went to a loud patient and told him to shut up. Obviously, the patient couldn't help it and had difficulties, but I couldn't take it anymore.

I was 18 at the time. I was one of the oldest patients on the unit. Typically, Cincinnati Children's only admits patients from ages 5 to 18. Some of the patients looked up to me because I was older. Some of the patients ran around the unit yelling. Some patients weren't being safe and would make lots of noise on the unit. I was told that I would feel better if I went to a different unit, but I felt like 2SW was the right place for me even though I wasn't as low functioning as the other patients. 2SW was a special unit within the hospital. The unit was mainly meant for children who have some sort of disability.

As I mentioned, there were groups. Mrs. Amber hosted an exercise group in which we would roll dice with a number. That number would be how many times we did toe touches, jumping jacks, or arm circles. Mrs. Amber taught me yoga and throughout my stay she helped me feel more comfortable in the unit.

Mrs. Amber listened to me and heard what I had to say. She helped me feel better when I was upset, or most importantly, sad. She educated me more on depression and what the signs and symptoms were. She spent a lot of time with me during my stay. Mrs. Amber took me off the unit a couple times to play basketball. She wanted me to reconnect with some old friends who I missed and hadn't talked to.

CHAPTER FOUR

We really didn't go too much into detail, but I did contact a couple friends when I was discharged. Mrs. Amber encouraged me to do so, so I did. I felt good about contacting friends from the past.

I learned many new things throughout my 50-day stay. I met so many nice people who helped me gain confidence and help lift my spirits so that I wasn't feeling down all the time. I would have times where I would laugh when I was engaged in conversations. I learned how to be in the moment and how to use my coping skills.

It's important to know that when you're going to be admitted, you'll be asked to have your blood drawn. For me, I didn't like blood draws. I refused the first time and became even more agitated when they came into my room telling me that it needed to happen. Fortunately, I didn't get my blood drawn that day. I was expected to have it done sometime during my stay. During my previous admissions, I would comply and get my blood drawn. Sometimes I would refuse, and they would do it on a day where I was feeling good because when I was agitated, my behavior was not right. Most times when I got agitated in the hospital, I would attack and destroy.

My blood pressure was checked often, and I had to get accustomed to this because I was in and out of the hospital. I would get really nervous when the staff took my blood pressure and my heart beats differently when I'm nervous. Thus, I would be diagnosed with high blood pressure the first time. Over time, I became less anxious with blood pressure readings and my blood pressure would normalize.

I would feel isolated and bored at points. I would just lay in my bed for a while having negative thoughts. Negative thoughts were often frequent and hard to control. I know now that negative thoughts are one of the major problems related to my depression. I learned new things that help with my negative thoughts such as new coping skills and being in the moment.

I started to get more comfortable about being in the hospital after each admission. I began to know the process already after my first couple admissions. Since I'd been to the hospital so many times, I learned how to control my behavior. I learned about time and patience while in the hospital. Patients who go to the hospital the first time would request to go home as I did. Patients need to realize that if you go to the inpatient unit, you will be expected to be responsible and follow the treatment plan in order to be discharged.

On the unit, I was able to make phone calls. I called my mother often, mostly upset. I thought she wouldn't let me come home and I was never going to be discharged. There was a day I got so angry that I ripped the phone off the wall. I wrote in my journal, "Ripping the phone off the wall won't help me in any way." (10/4/18) I was now supposed to use a conference phone in the conference room so that I wouldn't break the phone again if I got upset.

On the unit, there was a lunchroom. During certain parts of the day, there was a snack time. I would always get Cheetos and cookies. As you can imagine, spending 50 days in the hospital, I could eat Cheetos every day, which I did. I was introduced to Coke and Sprite later on in my stay. Mr. Okama and Shawn would let me have soda. I felt like there were some things I earned as I was 18 and thought I should be treated as an adult.

I attended IOP groups every Wednesday when I was an inpatient. Dr. Shaffer and Dr. Debra taught me many new things that I used personally when I was in the hospital. I learned about breathing exercises, how to make friends, and all this information I was given was great. I would go downstairs with my MHS and I would participate in the groups.

I met Mrs. Maddie, who is a Child Life specialist. She brought many coloring books and activities onto the unit. The activities weren't really exciting, but I enjoyed being around Mrs. Maddie. Later on, in my life, I was an intern for Child Life at the base hospital. I never saw Mrs. Maddie though because she was over at the College Hill campus, which was where I was admitted for all my hospitalizations. Mrs. Maddie would help me stay calm through my blood draws. Before my hospitalizations, I would pass out whenever I got my blood pressure taken. The sense of getting medical treatment would make me feel anxious and I would lose myself in the moment and pass out and throw up. Till this day, whenever I have to get an IV, I pass out. Other simple things I became comfortable with such as an EKG, blood pressure, and monitors. Mrs. Maddie would help me feel more comfortable so that I don't pass out or throw up.

When I woke up every morning, I grabbed towels and hospital clothes from the cabinets and brought them to my room. If you're admitted to a hospital you will be watched closely, and I was watched even when I was taking a shower. The workers didn't need to come into the bathroom, but I had to leave my door open. I was being watched to make sure I was being safe. My whole hospitalizations have been mainly about being safe and my care manager, Kris, made sure I was safe at all times even when I walked out of the hospital.

I had moments where I would become agitated and destroy property. I would rip certain things off the wall, I would throw my chair around in my room and make lots of noise. I wasn't being safe at all. I was so angry all the time, but I had some good moments and learning opportunities that helped me grow and become more familiar with life. These hospitalizations were life changing and I learned so much about reality and becoming an adult. If I didn't have these moments in my life, I wouldn't be here.

I worked on myself every day. I was always involved, and I participated. I never stayed in my room all day. I would come out of my room every morning and talk in groups. I would talk with other patients who were younger than I was. I gave some of the patients advice and for the patients who were non-verbal, I would communicate with them. I did cuss out some patients, but with most patients, I would smile and say hello. I liked to talk as much as I could because I didn't want to go through the stay alone. Anyone that is admitted should participate no matter what your condition is. Throughout my stay, I had nothing but support. There were a couple of rude people, but that didn't stop me from getting better and improving my mental health.

I learned more about confidentiality and respecting the privacy of others. When I was an inpatient and outpatient at Children's, I would meet new patients that come and go. I met some nice patients and some rude patients. I've had a couple of patients that tried to fight me. In addition, there were rules that I had to follow. Every day was structured and there would be shift changes and the float pool would change. I had some new staff that showed up, but most days I would hang out with Mr. Okama and Mr. Shawn.

After spending 50 days in the hospital, I was notified that I was going to be discharged. I was kind of confused and was super excited to leave. Like I said, I never thought I was going to be discharged. I was reminded that my stay was only temporary. I packed up all my stuff and waited a couple hours for my dad to come get me. I ripped off the sheets and blankets on my bed and put them in the hamper. Once I got ready to leave, I said goodbye to my staff. Not all of my staff that I worked with were there, but some were. I was escorted downstairs and out of the hospital. I got in the car and started crying. After all I've been through for 50 days and everything that went down, I was finally able to walk out of the hospital.

My experiences on 2SW still remain with me today. I still think about what I did and how I did it. I won't forget my stay on all the units I was on. I definitely won't forget my stay on 2SW.

Chapter Five
Last Resort: Electroconvulsive Therapy (ECT)

As I discussed previously, I was probated by the court with urgency because my doctor had prescribed electroconvulsive therapy treatments (ECT), and I was not agreeable. Although I have never had ECT before, I didn't like the topic or the way I had become a candidate for this treatment. After viewing YouTube videos and completing research on ECT, I was scared.

ECT is a procedure done in the morning. The patient is given general anesthesia and a muscle relaxant intravenously and electrodes are placed on the scalp. The thought of having an IV placed in my arm made me so ill I had to receive an intramuscular injection of ketamine before having my IV placed. I wasn't aware of the electrodes or the IV being placed in my arm. The doctor then passes a small electric current through the brain, intentionally triggering a brief, 30-second to 1-minute convulsion. ECT seems to cause changes in brain chemistry, which may quickly reverse symptoms of certain mental health conditions. After I awakened, the IV was removed, my family helped me dress, and I was taken to the car via a wheelchair. I remained drowsy for several hours afterward. Sometimes I experienced nausea. I completed these treatments three times a week for six treatments.

I was admitted in October and a week into my stay, I went into a conference room and my whole treatment team, which included my doctor, mother, father, social worker, and even some of my teachers from school were conferencing on the phone. I was hoping the meeting was related to discharge planning. Instead, my doctor provided education to me about ECT and the positive effects the treatment can have on depression. He also spoke about my medications being ineffective in battling my depression and suicidal ideation. Weaning from the Effexor was going to be a necessity in order to determine the effectiveness of the ECT treatments. This process would take about four weeks. After hearing this update, I became agitated, cursing, and completely confused as to how my life had become so out of control.

The probate court process was very challenging, as was the weaning process. Tremors, agitation, restlessness, and sadness were all feelings and behaviors I thought I came here to treat but now were much worse. The doctor said to be patient and ECT will help.

I had been admitted so many times to the point that nothing was working, and I needed something to help with my depression. This treatment required that I wean off of my medications, get blood drawn, and have an EKG so that in the upcoming weeks, I could have ECT done.

Once the day came for ECT, I woke up early in the morning around 6 a.m. My nurse, Mrs. Tina, gave me some medicine to help keep me calm during the procedure. I couldn't drink or eat anything before the ECT treatment. I was put onto a stretcher and put into the back of an ambulance. I had my blood pressure taken on the way to UC Health. I wrote an entry in my journal before my first ECT treatment, "There's nothing more powerful than emotions. I feel the saddest I have ever been in my entire life." (10/13/18) When I arrived at UC Health, I was very sad. I didn't want anything like this to happen to me, and I was minutes away from my first procedure. I was wheeled into same-day surgery and I was admitted into room 24 where I removed my hospital clothes and put on a hospital gown. On my feet I was required to wear non-skid brown socks. I waited on the hospital bed for the doctor to follow up with me. In the meantime, the nurse was asking me questions related to depression score and how my mood has been. I also completed memory work identifying pictures and I would repeat numbers in a sequential order. I was able to get settled in, but I didn't know what was going to happen next.

I was taken in an ambulance with my MHS, Mr. Shawn. He and I worked on a journal topic for things I wanted to remember prior to having my first ECT treatment. I was afraid that I would wake up and not remember anything like names or faces. I feared my brain would be swept clean. My care manager, Kris, was also there to help and support me through my first ECT treatment. I had no idea what to expect but as I became more familiar with the treatments, I realized that my memory would still be intact.

CHAPTER FIVE

The doctor and nurses walked into my room looking like they were about to start the treatment. I looked at my mom when she was talking to me. On the other side of the bed, I looked behind and saw a needle and the nurse began to inject me with the ketamine. I became upset and was being held down. I noticed everything turned dark and the people talking to me had deep voices. The deep voices were saying, "You're going to be ok, Daniel." It was almost like they were imaginary voices and at the same time I thought it was somebody trying to talk to me. This was very hard for me to go through. I've never experienced anything like this, and I wished others wouldn't have to be put in the position I was in.

I fell asleep and everything went black. Fifteen minutes later my nurse and mother woke me up. They asked me questions about if I remembered my name, if I knew where I was, and if I was having pain. I was so relieved that I had awakened. I remember saying, "Is it over yet? Thank goodness." I then fell back to sleep. My mother said this happened several times before we left the hospital.

The worst part of ECT was getting the ketamine injection into my deltoid muscle. I got used to the injection over time, but the ketamine medication hurt so bad when it was injected into my deltoid muscle. In order to receive general anesthesia and muscle relation musculation, I was required to have an IV and that couldn't happen without the ketamine injection first.

Almost every ECT treatment I had, I would write in my journal about how I felt before and after. Once the procedure was done, I wrote, "This part of my life is a lesson and a time to learn from and reflect on." (10/13/18) I thought ECT was a one-time thing and my parents and everyone I talked to never mentioned that I would repeat ECT a certain number of times. I didn't realize that I needed at least seven more treatments of ECT. When I returned back to the children's hospital, I was brought back up to the unit on a stretcher. I was so weak and dizzy that I needed help getting into my bed. Sometimes I needed medication for nausea or a headache after my return to the psych unit.

Two days later, I woke up again at 6 a.m. and got ready to head over to the UC Health Hospital. I wrote before my third procedure, "I am upset, I have five more treatments and they really hurt. This is not fair." I felt so angry and disappointed in myself that I had to be put through this. After having multiple ECT treatments, my whole body was aching, and I was still shaking with tremors caused by weaning off my medication. The ketamine injections hurt so much that I didn't want them anymore. After my sixth ECT treatment, I talked to the doctor and told him I was feeling much better but that I couldn't take any more treatments. I was done.

My short-term memory and concentration were somewhat worse immediately following ECT but currently, both have improved. According to research I had completed, memory loss and decreased concentration are common side effects of the ECT treatments. I felt good about journaling important things before my ECT treatments were initiated and I strongly encourage anyone who may be undergoing ECT treatments to journal their important thoughts or memories.

Although I strongly fought and resisted treatment, later on I realized the ECT treatments helped me. I can say now that I am better mentally because of the treatments. I can't imagine what would have happened if I didn't get help. I wouldn't be here. I would have taken my life. After I completed all my treatments, I was getting ready to return home. I was still having suicidal ideation and depression, but I was discharged once again. My suicidal ideation and depression were still haunting me, so the doctors initiated oral antidepressants. I didn't know it then, but I would undergo nine more treatments two months later. Those treatments made all the difference in the world. I completed those on an outpatient basis.

When I was discharged from the hospital in October, I was leaving behind relationships and memories I won't soon forget. After being on that unit for 50 days I had grown close to many healthcare providers. They provided friendship, hope, and encouragement to me over a long time period of time. I learned way more about my major depression and my treatments, but I also learned a lot about becoming an adult and managing my emotional self.

Once I got home, I was improving and doing way better than 50 days earlier. I knew that I didn't really want to end my life, but I was still

CHAPTER FIVE

dealing with depression. A couple months later I was admitted again. This was my final admission. I had an IOP (intensive outpatient program) group at Children's and when I finished with my group, I was escorted up to unit 3 South. I wasn't feeling worse than I was during my last admission. I didn't want to hurt myself or anything. I was just dealing with depression and anxiety.

I had to sign papers and do paperwork to be admitted again. Mr. Benjamin, whom I knew from my previous admissions, helped me get settled in. Some of the patients on the unit remembered who I was and so did the staff. I had worked with many of the staff on unit 3 South before. Some of the staff were disappointed to see me on the unit again. I just needed to get better.

My treatment team met, and I was included as usual and together we decided I would complete nine ECT treatments. I was agreeable at this point and would initiate the first treatment while in the hospital. I was disappointed in myself. I was currently a senior in high school and trying to complete all the coursework necessary to graduate. A teacher at the hospital would bring the laptop daily and I continued to work online. I was only an inpatient for two weeks. I had nine ECT treatments, most of which were on an outpatient basis and I did it voluntarily. My mother and father would take me in and take me home. Even though the ketamine injection hurt, it was able to get me through the treatments. I completed all nine treatments so at the end of the day I could feel better and safer. This was my last admission. Here I am. One year later.

Will I return to a happy life? You never know where life leads you. This was a learning experience and I definitely learned so much through Cincinnati Children's. I won't forget my five admissions and all the people who helped me through this rough path. If you helped me, talked to me, or made a situation better for me, I thank you.

Chapter Six
One Year Update: May 2020

Here I am, May 16, 2020. It has been a year since I completed my ECT treatments. I have come a long way. I am improving. I struggle with some depression and anxiety, but I am not like I was two years ago. I have occasional suicidal ideation; I am not shaking, and I am less agitated. I am 20 now, and since I am considered an adult, I am excluded from Cincinnati Children's hospital services. I have visited the Psychiatric Emergency Services (PES), which is part of University Hospital, when I have had suicidal issues.

The experience of going to PES was much different than Cincinnati Children's because the patients are older and deal with psychiatric issues that appear to be much worse than what I ever saw at Children's. The patients there would be yelling, strapped to stretchers, almost tipping them over, and using inappropriate language. The nurses and doctors always told me I didn't belong there. The caregivers were very kind and listened to my concerns, so I always went home.

My high school counselor provided me with an opportunity to attend Project SEARCH because I was diagnosed with ASD. My ASD is considered a disability and provides me with many useful community resources. Project SEARCH provides skills training so that I could be employable in a workplace as well as internships for individuals with disabilities. This program usually begins the year after high school. I accepted my high school diploma one year after I graduated because I was accepted into Project SEARCH, which started at the beginning of August 2019. Project SEARCH originated at Cincinnati Children's Hospital and now has program sites throughout the United States. The main goal is to educate and employ people with disabilities.

Before the actual training began, I purchased my metro access badge and then learned how to ride the metro bus. This was a new experience for me but my skills trainer, Amy, who spent time with me showing me the route, was very helpful. I rode with Amy three times before I rode independently. I would wake up every morning at

5:30 a.m., get dressed, and drive to Montgomery to catch the metro. I later on became more fluent with my routine. After several weeks of classroom learning, my instructor, Tina, discussed and delivered our internship assignments. We would have three internships during our school year.

Each internship I had lasted ten weeks. I became familiar with the Cincinnati Children's base location over time and I was doing well at this point in my life. I knew I had changed from wanting to hurt myself and I became successful. My first internship was in the Child Life department at Children's. I really enjoyed working with my managers and coworkers. The work I did was very rewarding and made me feel good inside. After ten weeks, I went on to interview in the teen health center. They hired me and my role was to clean and stock patient rooms. I really enjoyed working with the nurses and doctors. This was a great experience. After ten weeks, I interviewed for my last internship in Disabilities Services. I was hired and worked there in that department for only three weeks. A deadly virus, called the Coronavirus, struck Ohio. All non- essential workers were then required to stay at home. However, while interning, I worked in a database, helped organize the office, and completed some data entry tasks I was given. I was disappointed when the Corona virus became an issue, but I knew this wasn't the end because I still interacted with my classmates on Zoom.

During my time in Project SEARCH, I learned how to be professional, how to do well in an interview, and many other important life skills. I would recommend Project SEARCH. I was able to see some of the staff I had when I was on 2SW while interning at Children's. I was excited to see who I might stumble upon at Children's based on my past history. I also learned new things about myself. I gained social skills and I had great managers. I had nice classmates and job coaches who helped me during my internships. All my classmates and I were quarantined at home, so our graduation was completed online. The video was really nice, but I missed the opportunity to have a celebration with my classmates in person. Currently, I am still in touch with my classmates via social media.

CHAPTER SIX

I like rap and hip-hop music. I make beats and songs. I am going to release an EP. On my EP, there will be seven songs. I am hoping that I can show off my talent and create music for other people to listen to.

I hope that I can get my driver's license soon, so I can drive. I am also looking forward to buying my own apartment when I get older. After all the traumatic events I was put through, I am coming out striving and doing better than I ever have before. I have a great support team who are willing to make sure I do well and stay safe.

I have staff who I hang out with when my mom is working. After all I went through, I have to be supervised so that I am staying safe. I play basketball at LA Fitness with my staff; Ammar and I go places. I am hoping to move into being more independent and focusing on my own place sometime in the future.

I visit my dad every once in a while. In December, I took a flight down to Florida. I stayed at a trailer park with my dad and went fishing, and we went places such as the aquarium. I plan on going to Vermont to visit my dad again, hopefully this summer. My dad grew up in Massachusetts and has a house in Vermont. When I was younger I went skiing at Mount Snow and I visited places like Boston and Rhode Island.

I also like to visit my grandparents in Sandusky, Ohio. I was born in Sandusky. I moved to Cincinnati in 2008. When I was in Sandusky, I would go to the bay and hang out at Lake Erie next to Cedar Point. I had some good times when I was younger. I didn't want to leave Sandusky. I was sad that I left, but over time that sadness faded away.

I felt a different type of sadness later on in high school and that's when my depression started to kick in. All the traumatic events I went through changed me and I still think about the issues I was having. Depression has left a huge impact on me and I still struggle at some points. It's important that I learned how to deal with depression. There's always going to be a way out, but I made the decision to stay alive after what I went through. I choose life.

It's June 16. About a week ago, I was in the hospital for an attempt. I had been doing so well but I knew that I was going to make a move that wasn't going to be good. I attempted suicide.

It was a normal day. I got up and went to a group I had from 11 a.m. until 12 p.m. As I was in the car on my way home, I wasn't really feeling too good. Once I got home, I went inside and just felt like I wanted to do "something" because I felt like I wasn't getting enough help. I went into my mom's room and opened up the drawer. I found five small pills of Zyprexa and my night pills that I take before bed. So, I took all of the pills that were not locked up and went into my room and called 911.

I wasn't thinking right, and I was impulsive. I never wanted to end up back in the hospital, but I knew this time I was going to have some things done that I don't like. I was in the ambulance and I knew I was going to be alright, but I also knew that I wouldn't like the outcome. I was taken to the UC Health Hospital. Once I got situated and changed into my hospital clothes, I began worrying that I would have to get an IV. Before my ECT treatments I had expressed that I didn't like Ivs, and that I wouldn't be able to handle one. The nurse was ready to put the IV in, but I told her to wait a second. I then passed out for a couple seconds and threw up on myself. Everything went black; then I was helped back up. The nurse decided that if I can't do an IV, I would need a couple blood draws. So that's what we did.

The doctor called poison control and checked my levels. I was doing well and knew that I wouldn't have any issues regarding my physical health. I laid in my bed and was notified that I needed to stay eight hours to be cleared to enter the psychiatric unit at PES. My mom was notified by the police officer and she arrived at the hospital emergency room to stay with me until I was transported to PES. I waited and watched some TV in my bed. Once eight hours passed, I wasn't sure how much longer I would have to wait. I was also worried that I might have to spend a couple days on the psychiatric unit. I was disappointed in myself and felt guilty. I don't know what my life holds, but I know I have plenty of time to live. I just want to work on myself and get better. I want to live and explore but I can't do that

CHAPTER SIX

if I am visiting the hospital every month, and this time attempting suicide will definitely hold me back.

Once I was transported to PES, which was around 2:30 a.m., I went inside and met with a man who told me to sit somewhere on the unit. This night, I only got one hour of sleep. I was up waiting for the doctor and wondering what my next move might be. When everybody on the unit started waking up and people started moving around, I just sat and waited. The patients I was surrounded by just wanted to go home. Some wanted help and were asking for the nurse. I just sat and watched.

Next thing I know, in the morning this patient got up and started making a scene. I witnessed this man get put in restraints TWICE. I sat and watched from a couple feet away. This was slightly traumatic for me because I was personally put in restraints two years ago. I knew the feeling and anger that this patient had. It was tough because as a patient you have no control over anything. It seems as if the staff can do what they want when they're given a reason. Some staff were laughing, which I thought wasn't right. I just couldn't believe what I was seeing on the unit.

Once I met with the doctor, I expressed that I was safe and ready to go home. I didn't want to witness any more restraints or patients that aren't mentally right. I knew that this place wasn't for me. So, the doctor told me to call someone to come pick me up. I called my mom, and she was already waiting for me. I changed into my clothes and was discharged. I went back home feeling better.

Today, I still am not 100% mentally stable. I still make bad decisions. I don't want to go back to the hospital. I've been there at least 15 times and it's time for me to get better. It's a slow process but I believe in myself. I can do this!

It's July 19 and I am doing well at this moment. I recently quit my job at Kroger. I am going to look for a new job with the help of Tricia from OOD. I decided that I needed to quit working at Kroger because of my stress level and because it wasn't the right job for me as of right now. Time is quickly passing, and I continue to do well. I have had no more suicide attempts. I play a lot of basketball now almost every day; I am working on my vertical jump again. I see my new therapist once a week and I go to groups on Tuesdays and Wednesdays. I am working on my mental health. I have seen an improvement. I am hoping that in August I will be able to visit my dad in Vermont. I still have a lot to look forward to.

Chapter Seven
Depression and Suicide: The Reality

I have had my own suicide attempts and I think about how I could've ended my life. I am proud to say that I am still here today, living. Many who do not make it and commit suicide often tend to have a trigger or reason why they took their life. For me, I wanted to take my life because I had bad relationships, I felt disappointed in myself, and I was sad all the time reflecting on the past and what I went through. Others may experience what I have. As of right now, the coronavirus has led to more suicides. Many people may have lost their jobs, or they lost their homes and businesses. Mark Reger, PhD, chief of psychology services at the VA Puget Sound Health Care System in Seattle, says suicide is preventable. Suicide safety plans consist of recognizing warning signs or triggers of a developing crisis, learning coping strategies, and reaching out for help by calling the suicide hotline.

Suicide is the 10th leading cause of death in the U.S. In 2018, 48,344 Americans died by suicide. On average, there are 132 suicides per day. The rate of suicide should be a wake-up call. Many individuals that deal with depression, anxiety, or suicidal ideation should get professional help. Personally, I see a therapist, I attend groups, and I take medication to help with my depression and anxiety. When I was in the hospital, I learned a lot and I took those skills that I learned and incorporated them into my daily life. If someone is out there that needs help, they should be provided with help because it's difficult to see someone take their life. I really thought about it myself. I either get help or I take my life. I choose life because at the end of the day, I have family and friends that care about me and support me. If someone is going through depression, they deserve help. Those people who have lost their loved ones or don't have support at all need to be identified and helped through their struggles.

Depression is the leading cause of disability in the United States among people, ages 15 through 44. Two-thirds of people with depression do not actively seek nor receive proper treatment. Treatment is very important. I have had ECT treatment and other treatments as well when I was in the hospital. People who are admitted are usually in the hospital from 7-10 days, if not longer. It's important that each individual gets the right treatment and leaves the hospital feeling better. When I left the hospital 15+ times I wasn't 100% better, but I was feeling somewhat safer, even though I was re-admitted 7 times.

I want people to know that there is a light at the end of the tunnel. You may not like where you are right now as a person, but you will get better. I got better myself. I may not feel 100% better but at least I am able to say that there are things in life that I enjoy. Life shouldn't be miserable. Every person enters the world as a unique creation, and suicide shouldn't be how you leave. You can close your eyes and never wake up. Or, you can reach out like I did, and live many more years here with the blessings that God has given you.

When I visit my therapist and groups, I talk a lot about my past. I mention my hospital admissions and my history of depression. I was so sad at age 17 and 18, but I don't feel sadness as much anymore. I remember that sadness and that dark point in my life. Depression was controlling my life as I have mentioned before. One thing I mention that sticks out to me is, "How far will I make it in life?" Sometimes I don't believe in myself and my thoughts are filled with darkness. I don't see myself making it past a certain age because of my depression, suicidal thoughts, and actions. I want to live, knowing that I won't die to suicide. I want to tell myself that I can live forever, and I can make it past 100. I don't want to end my life at 22 or 50. I want to live as long as I can.

One quote that I found says, "Depression is like a war: you either win or die trying." I fight myself and beat myself down every day. I just want certain areas of my life to end. I wish I could go back and change my opportunities and chances that I had. I had no idea what depression was at age 15. I was living through depression for a long time.

I was diagnosed with major depressive disorder at 17. This diagnosis is described as the persistent feeling of sadness or loss of interest, including changes in sleep, energy levels, concentration, daily behavior, and self-esteem. Personally, I was noticing agitation and I was sleeping for a long time. Most days, I didn't want to get out of bed and go to school. I was missing the school bus a lot and I stayed home. When I went to school, I could only make it to three bells, then I would go to the school psychologist and express how I was feeling. I would leave school and go home crying a lot and I felt sad for hours laying in my bed.

I would write journals even before I was admitted my first time. On 1/30/17, I wrote, "I feel like I walked into another dimension. A new city or place—as if I am not going to ever see my friends again. This week I am not going to school for a full week due to what is happening throughout my life as a 16-year-old." I wrote, "I can only get through two bells, five at the most and then I crash."

I kept distant from friends and never communicated with them. I felt like over time I lost connections, and some unfollowed me on social media. I felt like I didn't get the chance to talk with someone who could've been my best friend because of depression, anxiety, and autism. I was so overwhelmed, and I had a dark cloud over my head every day. Now, as you're reading this, I hope you can understand what I was going through. I ignored a lot of people and I missed my opportunities, but I know that I wasn't in a good place and I hope that those of you reading can understand as well.

As my depression got worse, I was feeling like I needed to give up and end my life. I was socially crashing and burning. I was guilty of lying. I was spending more time sleeping and crying. I was isolating myself from the world. I went MIA. One day, I showed up to school after my hospital admission and one of my friends asked where I had been because I basically missed my whole senior year of high school. Everyone was talking about me and asking where I've been. Some thought I dropped out. Fortunately, I was still able to graduate through Aves Academy.

I would feel like I was hiding under a rock for a while. I would see my friends months later and they looked different. I was away from school for a while. I caught up with some people at graduation rehearsal and some people were surprised to see me. I felt like if I would have ended my life, I would have left a lot of people. I think about that a lot, almost every day. Many friends found out where I have been. Some never contact me anymore. I recently went to Weller Park to meet up with 4k and some people to play basketball. I saw some friends I haven't seen in a year. I can only imagine where we will be 50 years later. I sometimes wonder if I would be able to communicate with old friends from school. I let depression take me down a different path. It was a sad and dark path, but this was all a learning experience.

Chapter Eight
Mental Health: Positive Coping Skills

As I would struggle and face challenges, I would use my coping skills. Basketball has always been my favorite sport. I started playing at a young age, and till this day I continue playing. I grew up watching LeBron play on the Cavaliers. I wanted to ball like LeBron, and I would add his form and step back into my game.

As I would go through a tough time in life, basketball was one thing that helped me get through my depression. Luckily, Children's Hospital had an inside basketball court that I would play at when I got to go off the unit. My last admission, I lost interest in basketball. I started playing again later on in 2020. Ammar, my friend, has gotten me out of the house and onto the basketball court and now, I am playing basketball once again.

I was on lots of basketball teams throughout my time and I played my freshman year in high school. I stopped trying out for the team and focused more on my mental health. I played guard and I was in the post most times. I didn't start but I would play a decent amount of time.

When I played in the rec league, I would dominate. I was mainly a defensive player. I was working on my vertical jump and later on in high school, I learned to dunk. I would use my vertical to get rebounds and block shots. I was in a dunk contest during a pep rally. I felt embarrassed because I couldn't get off the ground like the other contestants. No matter that, I won the contest from a one-handed dunk with an alley-oop. Everyone was cheering. I was super excited, and this was the happiest moment of my time in high school.

High school was very hard to get through, but I had my coping skills and I had people that supported me. I went to groups located at the high school during my lunch break and after school as well. I wanted to fit in and going through school was a learning experience. My coping skills, such as writing, playing basketball, listening to and making music, and walking would help put my feelings to the side and these skills I had would help me focus on being in the moment.

Basketball has helped me grow as a person. I made friendships and I practiced this sport every day to make the basketball team. I worked hard and I felt happy and till this day basketball brings me happiness. No matter what you go through, you will have something that makes you feel good. Anyone that goes through depression, anxiety, or if you have any disability, you should find that one thing that makes you feel good. For me, basketball is what makes me feel better during a tough situation. I will continue to play basketball. Coping skills are important in life.

As I mentioned, I not only like to listen to music, but I like to make music myself. I have released music on iTunes and other major streaming platforms. Music also helps me get through tough times. I like all kinds of music. I mainly enjoy rap music the most, but I like to listen to 80's music and old tunes. Some of my favorite artists are Frank Sinatra, Drake, SET Meech, Mac Miller and Mundo. Some of my favorite artists have died from overdosing, and I think about how blessed I am to still be here. Music is powerful and certain artists leave effects on people with how they sing/rap in their songs.

I know a lot about music. I have my own microphone, interface, and monitors. I've helped produce and mix music and I like to give feedback to other artists within the city. I like to listen to certain songs on repeat and I listen to music to help me fall asleep.

When I was in the hospital, I would play music almost every day. I would request songs to play during groups and other times when I was sitting outside of my room. I would write lyrics with some of my staff and they would tell me how good an artist I am. I felt like my music could help people vibe and most people would support my music.

Chapter Nine
Set Back: September 2020

Here I am, on September 29, 2020, I am continuing to progress. Last Wednesday, September 23, I had a setback. I was doing well, and I had my depression group earlier in the day at Ikron. Once I got home, I was watching TV until my mother returned home from work. I was having lots of anxiety later in the day and I ended up dialing 911, hoping to get help. I waited for the police to show up, and I told them how I was feeling. I didn't want to let anyone down and I felt like getting help was my best option even though I want to stay out of the hospital.

I was taken to Bethesda North Hospital in the police car, where my mother works as a Registered Nurse (RN). My mother was sleeping when I called 911. The officer walked in and told my mother that I would be taken to the hospital. The officer who took me to the hospital made me feel better about the situation and told me that if I ever need someone to talk to, I can call him. When I got to Bethesda North, I walked in and everyone was looking at me and I felt slightly intimidated. I was given a pink slip and was told that I would have a 72-hour hold. I was taken to an open bed in the ER. I got settled in and I immediately saw the nurse. I was told that I would need to have an IV and they needed to take blood. I told the doctor and nurse that I cannot handle Ivs, so they agreed to just take my blood instead.

I ended up staying in the ER overnight and my mother was, once again, by my side. Once I woke up the next day, I waited till noon and was told that I would be transferred to a psych unit. I've never heard of this hospital but was hopeful that in the upcoming days, I could get through an inpatient stay successfully. The EMTs entered my room, and I was put onto a stretcher and was escorted out to an ambulance. I was heading to the psych unit and was being asked questions. I've been feeling better. but I knew that I would be inpatient for a couple days. Once I got to the psychiatric unit, I entered and noticed that the staff and patients were not wearing masks. I was told that I would not need to do a swab test for Covid-19. Other hospitals require a swab test but the psychiatric unit I went to did not require it, which I was happy about because I don't like going through that process.

I got settled in and communicated with the nurse on the unit. I was asked a couple questions such as, "Do you want to hurt yourself or others?" I was also asked to do a skin check to see if I cut myself anywhere. Once I completed my questions with the nurse, I walked to the concourse area of the unit and watched TV. The patients I was with throughout my five-day stay were inpatients because of drug problems and homelessness. Some other patients were young and were dealing with the same issues I was having. I was shy in the beginning of my stay, as usual, but as each day went by, I was communicating more and more.

The staff I had were partially helpful. The staff tried to cheer me up and encouraged me to attend groups. Personally, I never missed one group and I was at breakfast, lunch, and dinner every day. The food I was given was decent. My favorite meal that I had was a cheese quesadilla and chile. Most patients complained about how bad the food was and how bad the hospital smelled. I didn't want to talk with any patients because I felt like they might ask me personal questions and I didn't want to affiliate myself into a situation that I didn't want to be involved in. My main goal was to learn how to communicate and take my PRN rather than being admitted again to the hospital. My support team encouraged me to give them a call whenever I need help or if I am having trouble with anything.

In the adult psych unit, I had a roommate and I would maintain good hygiene. I tried my best not to leave a mess because I've never had a roommate throughout my time on psych units. I wanted to keep a clean space and I would try my best not to be loud or anything that would wake my roommate from sleeping. I would use the shower in my room and the water spilled onto the floor and flooded the bathroom. I had this same experience on 2SW at Children's.

My mother bought me clothes and I finally received them three days into my stay. I was wearing a hospital gown previously but since I received my personal clothes, I wore those for the rest of my stay.

My clothes were not allowed to have strings due to hospital policies, which was a rule at every other hospital I've been to.

My experience in the adult psych unit was much different from Children's and I hope to never return as an inpatient but if I need to, I will. All that I've been through, I plan to now implement my resources such as calling my support team like doctors, my therapist, family, police officer, and my caregiver, Omar. I also know that a PRN would help to calm me down. I also like to implement my coping skills like music and basketball.

I can prevent hospital admissions; I can work on progressing and learning from my mistakes. Life isn't perfect and I will give my best effort every day. For however long I live, I want to make a difference. I know that writing my own story could help someone feel better or they could relate. I hope readers will learn and benefit from my story. I would like to give thanks to all the people who supported me throughout these past three years. It's been a long road, and I hope to see many more years ahead.

Chapter Ten
A Mother's Perspective – Julie Nardi

"For I am the LORD, your God, who takes your right hand and says to you, Do not fear; I will help you." Isaiah 41: 13

Care, love, lonely, overwhelming, helpless, angry, and proud are only some of the emotions I felt while raising Daniel and then again while assisting with his book. I recall the frequent tantrums and animal-like behaviors that seemed to last for hours, all the nights I had to lay in his bed until he fell asleep, and finally, the day I drove to Akron, Ohio, alone with Daniel to get him evaluated and diagnosed with autism. The diagnosis was something I expected but, at first, I did not want to accept it.

Ultimately, I wholeheartedly embraced the condition, and we began the journey. The journey was down a path wrought with darkness and sunlight, overgrowth and brush, but also with tools we were given to clear the path. We have met so many people along the journey, some are on it too, some just get in the way, but a few really want to guide and protect.

I believe the most important intervention was seeking help immediately for speech and socialization. Once Daniel was able to begin speaking and actually communicating what he needed or wanted the temper tantrums decreased. I became his "rock." His security blanket.

Going to visit friends/family was challenging as he wanted to be at home, "playing parking lot" with his Match Box cars. We had to have his cars with us everywhere we went. If someone wanted to play along or misalign the cars, look out for a tantrum.

Head Start helped a lot and then he started school with an IEP to meet his learning needs, as well as his speech needs. He had created a special language all his own. He used his special language at home, saying words in his own way, and we accepted it as "Daniel's way." The doctors told me Daniel would be unable to learn to read, but with the help and guidance of his special education teacher, Mrs. Kyle, he learned to read! I was so proud of him. The years that followed were more challenging. Intervention teachers saw him as handsome, strong, and capable. However, after one quarter they began to understand as his test scores plummeted and the comprehension of subject matter did not exist. Each year was the same; I had to intervene and question why the IEP was not being followed and then request numerous conferences, expressing concerns and validating his diagnosis of autism. The teachers would finally understand, but no collaboration occurred with the teachers for the next year. During his junior year of high school, I was forced to have a re-evaluation to prove his diagnosis. This cost $2500. And, of course, it did validate the diagnosis.

Daniel was to take a pre-ACT test in the auditorium where the entire class of approximately 650 students sat. The principal stood up and said, "All the students with accommodations please go to the teacher over there and you will go into a different room for your testing." How many students got up? None. Daniel heard students say, "What does that mean?" Then other students said, "Oh, that's for all the dumb kids." Daniel said, "I didn't get up. I didn't answer any of the questions. I didn't know what to do."

The doctors told me kids with autism don't usually do well on team sports, so when he took an interest in swimming I was pleased. He did very well. I was so nervous for him when he first tried out for basketball in fourth grade. He did not make the team. However, the coaches told him what he needed to practice, and he did every day. The following year he tried out and made the A team! I cried. He smiled. He stayed focused and played alongside the same boys for four years. Four happy years of being included and not judged.

Simple things happened in high school, causing traumatic breakdowns. Friends matured, girls became more interesting, Daniel started shaking because he was so nervous; he couldn't say anything right. Socially awkward. A coach left his information laying out, a teammate saw it and pretty soon everyone knew Daniel was autistic. Daniel asked me, "What does that mean, Mom?" One of the saddest days of my life. He knew. The blinders were off. I never kept it a

CHAPTER TEN

secret, but he understood that autism meant how his life may be affected. Depression followed.

He has written about this. I will say, I took him to the hospital, alone, every time. No one has been with me to support me. I have always been with Daniel. Watching him be placed in four-point restraints was devastating. I sobbed. He was very ill. I had been taking him to a psychiatrist and therapist, but he needed more help. Thus, our first admission of many to come.

Hearing my child say he "would be better off dead" is like someone socking me in the gut—hard. I was unable to catch my breath or stop crying. Revisiting all these times through this book has been just as difficult. However, I believe his stories and mine may be of help to someone or the many who might be struggling or looking for help. I searched and learned about services Daniel would qualify for such as Medicaid and disability services through Hamilton County. Loads of paperwork, but every bit of it was worth it. The case managers guided me and led me down the right path. All the while I prayed and prayed some more.

When ECT became the last resort, I figured out how to apply for guardianship and did it. We were all terrified of the procedure and what the outcomes would be. Thankfully, the outcomes were better than expected. Daniel's level of depression decreased. Just recently, I had to complete the guardianship report. I figured it out and did it. With Medicaid, there are many choices. I did not know this at first, so now I will be making a better selection in order that Daniel will have more choices for healthcare providers.

One of the most challenging issues of late is the unknown. Daniel may have a flare-up of depression at any given point. Triggers during this time of Covid-19 are many, and we are coping as best we can. However, I have missed work, and this creates financial instability for me. His caregivers and I work very closely together to manage these times. Recently, he was able to go into respite care because he has an IO waiver. I was very thankful for this. It meant he lived with another family for one week, allowing some distance for him to feel better and me to work. He has been able to learn new skills through

IKRON and to receive individual counseling from a therapist there too. OOD provides a designated number of paid hours for individuals to learn work skills.

Daniel has many interests and goals. I am here to encourage and cheer him on toward those goals. I am so proud of who he has become: a kind, thoughtful, hard-working young man. He feels compelled to share this story and truly believes this story will touch at least one person, and I believe many will realize they are not alone in their struggle and will have hope for the future.

Chapter Eleven
ASD: Signs/Symptoms/ Diagnosing and Treatment

Classification of ASD

According to the American Psychiatric Association's, *Diagnostic and statistical manual of mental disorders* (5th ed. Arlington, VA: American Psychiatric Association; 2013), Autism Spectrum Disorder, ASD, affects communication and behavior. Although autism can be diagnosed at any age, it is a developmental disorder because symptoms appear in the first two-to-three years of life. According to the *dsm/5 guide*, the standard used to diagnose mental disorders, individuals with ASD have:

1. Difficulty with communication and interaction with other people

2. Restricted interest and repetitive behaviors and

3. Difficulty functioning properly in school, work, and other areas of life.

Autism is known as a "spectrum disorder" because there is a wide variation in the type and severity of symptoms individuals experience (1).

Autism spectrum disorder includes conditions that were previously considered separate. These separate diagnoses included pervasive developmental disorder, Asperger's syndrome, childhood disintegrative disorder, and RETT syndrome (2).

Rather than characterizing these diagnoses, APA has adopted a dimensional post to diagnose disorders that fall underneath the autism spectrum umbrella. Some experts have proposed that individuals on the autism spectrum may be better represented as a single diagnostic category. Within this category, the *dsm/5* has proposed a framework of differentiating each individual by dimensions of severity, as well as associated features, "i.e. known genetic disorders and intellectual disability" (3).

Another change in the *dsm-5* includes collapsing social and communication deficits into one domain. Thus, an individual with an ASD diagnosis will be described in terms of severity of social communication symptoms, severity of fixated or restricted behaviors or interest, hyper or hypo sensitivity to sensory stimuli, and associated features. The restriction of onset age has also been loosened from 3 years of age to early developmental period, with a note that symptoms may manifest later when social demands exceed capabilities (4).

Signs and symptoms:

Autism spectrum disorder (ASD) is characterized by persistent challenges with social communication, social interaction, and by the presence of restricted, repetitive patterns of behavior, interest or activities (5). Possible red flags of ASD are a child does not respond to their name by 12 months of age, does not point at objects or show interest, avoids eye contact and wants to be alone, has delayed speech and language skills, repeats words or phrases over and over (echolalia), and gets upset by minor changes (6).

Diagnoses:

Diagnosing ASD can be difficult because there is no medical test, like a blood test, to diagnose the disorder. ASD can be detected as early as 18 months or even earlier in some cases (7). Ideally, the diagnoses of ASD should be given by a team of professionals from different disciplines, including child psychologists, child neurologists, and psychologists. This diagnosis should only be made after the child has been observed in many different settings (8). As of 2019, psychologists evaluating ASD would wait until a child showed initial evidence of ASD tendencies, then administer various psychological assessment tools. Among these measurements, the autism diagnostic interview and autism diagnostic schedule are considered the "gold standards" for assessing ASD (9). Various other questionnaires such as the childhood autism rating scale, autism treatment evaluation checklist, Peabody picture vocabulary test and the Peabody picture are typically attributed in the ASD assessment battery.

Causes:

While specific causes of ASD remain unclear, many risk factors identified in research may contribute to ASD. These risk factors include genetics, prenatal and perinatal factors, neuroanatomical, abnormalities, and environmental factors. Current research suggests that genes that increase susceptibility to ASD are ones that control protein synthesis in neuronal cells in response to cell needs, activity, and adhesion of neuronal cells, synapse formation and remodeling, and excitatory to inhibitory neurotransmitter balance (10).

Management:

Currently, no treatment has been shown to cure ASD, but several interventions have been developed and studied for use with young children. These interventions may reduce symptoms, improve cognitive ability and daily living skills, and maximize the ability of the child to function and participate in the community.

There are many types of treatments available. These include applied behavior analysis, social skills training, occupational therapy, sensory integration therapy, and use of assistive technology. The types of treatments generally can be broken down into the following categories: Behavior and Communication Approaches, Dietary Approaches, Medication, Complementary and Alternative Medicine (11).

Support Services

Cincinnati Children's Hospital Medical Center

Medicaid application

County DDS services

SSI benefits

IEP information

Metro services

Probate court in county of residence: Guardianship order

Electroconvulsive Therapy

Greater Cincinnati Behavioral Services

East Side Day Academy

Sources

(1). Lord C, et al (November 2000). "Autism spectrum disorder." NEURON. 28 (2); 355-63.

(2). Kulage Km, et al. "How will Dsm-5 affect autism diagnosis? A systematic literature review and meta-analysis." *Journal of Autism and Developmental Disorders.* 44 (8); 1918-32.

(3). Klin A (May 2006). "Autism and Asperger's syndrome: an overview." *Revista Brasileira de Psiq uiatria.* 28; S3-11.

(4). Dsm-5 diagnostic criteria. U.S. Department of health and US services. Interagency autism coordinating committee. (17) May 2017.

(5). Lord C, et, al. (August 2018). "Autism spectrum disorder." *Lancet.* 392 (10146); 508-520.

(6). "Signs and Symptoms of Autism Spectrum Disorders." *Centers for Disease Control and Prevention,* Centers for Disease Control and Prevention, 27 Aug. 2019, www.cdc.gov/ncbddd/autism/signs.html.

(7). "Autism spectrum disorder; screening and diagnosis." Centers for Disease Control and Prevention. 26 February 2015.

(8). Simms, MD. (February 2017). "When autistic behavior suggests a disease other than classic autism." Pediatric Clinics of North America. 64 (1); 127-128.

(9). Huerta, M, Lord C. (February 2012). "Diagnostic evaluation of ASD." Pediatric Clinics of North America. 59 (1); 103-11.

(10). Chen JA, et al (2015). "The emerging picture of ASD; genetics and pathology." *Annu Rev Pathol.* (10); 111-44.

(11). "Treatment and Intervention Services for Autism Spectrum Disorder." Centers for Disease Control and Prevention, 23 Sept. 2019, www.cdc.gov/ncbddd/autism/treatment.html.